Letters to HAE:
Finding Hope While Living
with Hereditary Angioedema

Kristy Brosz

Dedication

*For all HAE patients, caregivers, family members
and professionals.
Thank you to each of you for being brave enough to advocate
for a better understanding of living with HAE
in your own circle of influence.*

AND

*For the HAE patients who are now with us
only in spirit.
Thank you for your advocacy efforts in both
your life and your legacy.*

Table of Contents

Acknowledgements

There are many individuals who deserve thanks for turning this book into a reality. First and foremost, thanks to my remarkable family. Without all of you this story would not have been written. An extra special thanks to my extraordinary husband, John Brosz. I am so grateful to you every day for your many strengths that include: bravery, giant doses of love, remarkable courage, great sense of humour, an strong shoulder to cry on, creativity, and the ability simultaneously hold my fear while ensuring we build beautiful life for our family. Most of all, I'm extremely grateful for your never-ending ability to help me find the fluidity of hope in every challenge HAE bring us.

A very special thank you also goes to Dr. Tom Bowen for his ever-present advocacy mantra in the HAE community:

"It can be done, it must be done, for the sake of our patients."

I will forever be grateful for Dr. Bowen's ability hold onto hope to create a better quality of life for all HAE patients. I am so grateful for this his wisdom, determination, advocacy, expertise, and willingness to think outside the box to not only help me access home infusion, but to also help me live my best life possible every step of the way.

Finally, an additional thank you goes out to the many individuals within my own HAE advocacy community who have helped me find hope at various points on this journey: Julia Hews-Girard, Dr. Dawn Good Year, Morna Brown, Marie Cailes, Joanne Frizzel, Della Cogar Jacquie Badiou, Dr. Bruce Ritchie, CHAEN physicians, and all the past and present staff at the Southern Alberta Comprehensive Care Bleeding Disorders Clinic and FMC Day Medicine Clinic. Thank you to each one of you for your support, advocacy, and willingness to sit deeply in the HAE lived experience.

Preface
Hereditary Angioedema

This book is intended to relay my experience with the community of hereditary angioedema (HAE). It is not a professional medical guide outlining medical knowledge of this disorder and how it should be diagnosed, treated, and managed. However, for those readers that may not be familiar with HAE this section provides an overview of what HAE involves.

HAE is a genetic, chronic, rare blood disorder affecting 1 in 30,000 to 1 in 50,00 individuals. It is an autosomal dominant genetic disease associated with a deficiency or dysfunction of C1 esterase inhibitor (C1-INH).

HAE causes a spontaneous, recurrent, unpredictable, and potentially life-threatening swelling in soft tissues of the body, often causing severe pain. Swellings may be overtly seen in various parts of the body such as facial swelling (think of the face of boxer who has dramatically lost a boxing match) or an abdominal swelling that may swell similar to someone who looks as though they are carrying a full-term pregnancy. However, swelling may also not be visible at all, such as the life-threatening swelling of the esophagus that can lead to asphyxiation. Left untreated swellings often last for 3-7 days, causing many days of disability per year for those affected.

HAE swelling varies between individuals and even across an individual's life span. HAE is unpredictable in nature and therefore the frequency, severity, and type of each HAE swell does not predict the frequency, severity, and type of the next HAE swell. Knowledge of triggers for HAE swells are still very much an emerging area of understanding and may include, but are not limited to: specific medications; hormones; dental work; infections and/or medical procedures; repetitive motions; injuries; psychosocial stressors/overall stress; and any trauma to the body that would cause additional stress to the body.

HAE swellings often have a significant impact on the body in the affected area. They are extremely painful and can require significant time for convalescence depending on the area of the body inflicted. For example, an abdominal swell which may go on for several days not only causes extreme pain (pain akin to kidney stones, childbirth, or a bowel obstruction), but also vomiting, diarrhea, and associated medical concerns related to being unable to eat or drink over that time. In addition to recovering from this physiologically and psychologically traumatizing period, patients must also deal with extreme fatigue and specific side effects (for example, kidney stones may arise from these repeated periods of dehydration).

While there is no cure for HAE, the past decade has seen the development of seven treatment options for HAE. However, given the complexity of approval systems and immense cost of such treatments for this rare disorder, they are frequently not widely accessible to HAE patients across the globe. Even once patients are able to successfully win their battle to access treatment, there are often many barriers to treatment; a particularly problematic issues is the need for IV access for most treatment options. Home infusion has been a key delivery model in the treatment of HAE that allows patients and caregivers to treat their swellings at home as they occur and providing patients with much more control over their disease and a significant increase in their quality of life.

HAE patients are often misdiagnosed and/or undertreated for many years or decades due to:

- The many barriers to accessing appropriate comprehensive care for HAE;

- the lack of understanding of the disease with the medical and scientific community; and

- The overall rarity and unpredictable nature of HAE

- General complex nature of the pathways related to the C1-inhbitor deficiency or dysfunction.

However, within the last two decades, much progress has been made toward the diagnosis, prognosis, and treatment of HAE through dedicated advocacy efforts, clinical trials, and the development of international consensus guidelines. The development of these guidelines has seen international efforts to:

- reduce the lengthy time frame for diagnosis;
- establish standards for comprehensive care, including home infusion standards, and define interdisciplinary team roles;
- share findings from clinical trials; and
- develop several specialized protocols for treatment of unique populations of HAE patients.

Such immense progress in such a short time is truly remarkable and reflects key progress forward in the HAE community.

It is not the intent of this book to duplicate the information that has already been published in emerging areas for HAE. Nor is it the intent of this book to provide specific medical advice on treating or identifying HAE. Patients should always consult with their own medical professionals for further discussions on case specific diagnosis, treatment, and overall support. The intent of this book is to begin to address the psychosocial experience of HAE patients and caregivers.

Despite the gains in medical understanding and protocols for HAE, one key area has been left behind in the development of HAE support. This gap includes a solid understanding of trauma-informed psychosocial treatments and interventions along with advocacy for the emotional and psychosocial aspects of living with HAE.

Therefore, the purpose of this book is twofold:

1. To highlight the complex nature of the traumatic emotional and psychosocial impact of HAE for both patients and caregivers; and

2. To provide a call to action for psychosocial professionals to develop and enhance specific trauma-informed psychosocial interventions for patients and caregivers.

The book is divided into five sections that speak to key psychosocial considerations interwoven within the HAE community. Each section contains letters to HAE from a HAE patient. It then contains responses back to those letters from a caregiver.

For the purpose of this book, a HAE caregiver is any family member, friend, or other supporter that accompanies a HAE patient through their journey. At the end of each section is a toolkit with practical tips for HAE patients, caregivers, and professionals.

This book is not meant to be prescriptive; I hope to give a voice to those living with HAE and further the conversation. It is intended to provide a hopeful framework for living well with this disease regardless of where one may find themselves on their disease trajectory.

To find additional resources and to share your thoughts please visit my author website at: https://kristybroszauthor.weebly.com/.

Section I

Trauma & The Challenges of Living an Ultra-Rare Life

"The only victory that is gained through [illness] is a new perspective; the only defeat is giving into bitterness."
Mike Lang

Dear HAE,

All the medical literature written describes you as an "episodic" disease, but, today, you feel like a huge never-ending force in my life. You impact me every day in every way. You are far from episodic. You are a continuous disease.

Today you are too large to conquer, or even walk beside with any type of gentleness. You feel all-consuming and life-limiting. You bring me to my knees to the depths of despair. I rage against your influence on my life.

As with most challenges in my life, you inspire me to learn from you. In the past, if I listened quietly between the fear and pain, I found there were lessons to be learned. Perhaps if I make a conscious choice to listen to you again, I will find a way to live well on the other side of some of the darkness you bring me.

Therefore, HAE, I have decided to write to you to explore what it is you bring me. I hope to learn what lies on the other side of this intense challenge of living with you. You have coursed through my veins, filled my entire being, since before I was born. To help enhance my understanding of these lessons, my caregiver has agreed to answer my letters. The caregiver who has been my rock, the one beside me in all of this, who has been just as affected by you as I have. The one who witnesses the impact of HAE just as much as I have, but from outside of my body.

Perhaps, through exploring this journey together, we will be able to find the ever-elusive sense of hope that seems to have disappeared.

From,

The Searching HAE Patient

Dear Searching HAE Patient,

I also have times where the very force of HAE feels far too life-altering, defeating, and consuming. Therefore, I will write letters back to you in an attempt to further understand the lessons that ebb and flow on the continuum between fear and hope. And, in doing so, I hope to also gain understanding for myself.

I look forward to joining together to listen deeply in the dark places to find where hope has hidden. Perhaps we can encourage it to emerge.

From,

The Also Searching HAE Caregiver

Dear HAE,

Why are you raging again today? What did I do to set you off? I've gone through all my list of triggers and can't match your outburst to any of them. I've done everything right: taken all my meds and infusions on time; paced myself so I do not take on too much; ate healthy; went to bed early; avoided germs/infections; and tried to be gentle with myself to avoid additional stress. But when you woke me up, I had that familiar feeling of terror like my breath was being sucked out of me.

Apparently, you are trying to tell me that you have more lessons to teach me. You remind me that you, as a disease, vary so much between individuals. You remind me that you even varies within the same individual's lifetime. You remind me that the best thing I can do is just keep learning from each swell, from each experience. The harder I cling to the frustration and terror of it all, the less I can learn from it.

You also remind me that despite how it feels today, I'm not learning this in isolation. There are so many others learning right along with me: my support system; other HAE patients across the globe; my medical team; researchers; and the curious minds housed within pharmaceutical companies. We are all seeking wisdom to see what you are trying to each us.

However, for this moment, I will rage a little.

At how unfair you are.

At how you can dash my dreams for the future in an instant.

At how I wish you didn't exist.

At how you force me every moment of every day to try to make decisions that have no solid answers, only further questions.

At how your treatment options present such risks and have limited evidence bases simply because you are so ultra-rare. It is impossible to study you with large scale, international, double-blind trials like more common diseases have the luxury of including in their evidences bases.

At how you have produced such unpredictability throughout my life thus far.

At how you never appear the same between any two patients, even within my own family.

At how you force me to live an extraordinary life simply by requiring me to seek out creativity and tenacity to survive through another day.

At how often I have to make a conscious choice to not live in denial simply so I can literally live through each day.

At how much the advances in this disease are at the mercy of such complex systems such as blood banks, pharmaceutical companies, insurance companies, ethics boards, special authorization criteria, and many others that interplay between all these systems.

At how much I simply hate you with every part of my being.

And then I know I have to contain the rage, or you will become even larger than I know.

Therefore, instead, I will quiet my heart and mind as I am sure you have another lesson ready for me if I'm prepared to listen. So, I close my eyes and try to begin again with that mindset.

From,

Raging HAE Patient

Dear Raging HAE Patient,

I am here beside you also raging at what HAE has taken from all of us. You are correct in that you are not the only one learning; I've had to learn as well as we walk through this together. I have to learn in every moment of every day, just as you do.

I admit, today when you were not looking, I also raged at HAE.

I raged at how HAE brings you so much fear and pain that it makes you question your strength. For the record---you are stronger than you will ever know. Yet, I have witnessed how HAE can take that away in one swift moment, as soon as an HAE swell begins to surface.

I raged at how helpless us caregivers are when HAE strikes. I so desperately want nothing more than to take away your pain, fear, frustration, and multitude of losses to give you back what you have lost. However, I also realize I am powerless.

HAE is a burden that will never play fair and that is simply not acceptable.

I raged at how little others understand all that comes with this disease. They have no clue about what you face every day, just to keep breathing. I see how hard you try to reach your goals and dreams despite this terrible disease. It is not fair that so much of the world will never know the extent of the battles you have to face and how resilient you are.

I raged at how other medical professionals treat you. How they make such snap judgments because they have a medical degree. None of these decisions are based on you as a unique human being. Or, because they have gotten to know this ultra-rare disease with extremely variable clinical presentations, treatments, and life-long impact on the body.

I raged at the fact that what little control you have over your whole life can be taken away in an instant by such large, faceless, interconnected systems that know nothing about you as a person. They have no idea how one small action or decision can affect your entire life. They also have no idea how it also affects my entire life as well, as my head, heart, and soul attempts to carry this burden with you.

And then, through all the raging, I realized your calm approach to such difficulties is what is needed. To not give into the rage, but rather to search for the lessons on the other side of the rage. To not let the rage win.

Perhaps we need to rage together against this horrible disease for a time; but we shall not let it define us. Instead, let's sit and listen together as we search for what lies on the other side of the challenges.

From,

Also Raging HAE caregiver

Dear HAE,

I concede. You win today.

From,

The Defeated HAE Patient

Dear Defeated HAE Patient,

I know it's so hard.

Watching you struggle so much I feel defeated too.

Regardless of how defeated we both are, just know I'm here.

I will sit in the hard places with you.

From,

Also Defeated HAE Caregiver

Dear HAE,

Ditto to yesterday.

Why must you be so hard?

That is all.

From,

The Ultra-Defeated HAE Patient

Dear Ultra-Defeated HAE Patient,

I'm still here.

My heart feels defeated along with your heart.

However, I'm still sitting in the dark places with you.

I can't promise to take away the fear and pain, but I can promise I will be beside you regardless of how deep it goes. And I don't make promises I can't keep.

I'm here.

Always.

Carry on in the dark places and I'll be beside you.

From,

Also Ultra-Defeated HAE caregiver

Dear HAE,

Today I woke up determined to feel less defeated. I'm still wallowing from what you took from me these last few days.

It's hard to miss out on important aspects of my life due to your unexpected ways of infiltrating everything and adding one more loss.

This morning I can rationalize that, in the grand scheme, this one loss not so bad. Not really. But this loss doesn't exist in isolation. It's in addition to the layers of losses heaped up on top of each other over the course of my lifetime.

When I sit in the cumulative losses that HAE has brought me, it becomes far too easy to wallow in it all, to give up, and give in to a life of disability.

But as my dreams and plans for future pass before me, I also know that I desperately want to show HAE that it cannot win; while it will always be a part of my genetic code, it will not conquer my soul, heart and mind.

HAE, the whispers that you are sharing with me today are trying to remind me that your strength for imposing limitations on me is great and all consuming.

However, I have other intentions for the day. Therefore, today, I will likely take some time to listen to your whispers to find out how much you want to rage today. But I am determined that you won't fully win.

I have a purpose for the day, and I am going to fulfill it one way or another!

From,

The Determined HAE Patient

Dear Determined HAE Patient,

Thank you for sharing your strength to keep going. You have taken such difficult pain and loss and remain determined to get through another day.

I must admit that, when you were finally able to get some sleep after this last massive swell episode, I snuck away for a few minutes. I feel guilty that I did, but I needed time for me. I sat just far enough away so that you wouldn't see the tears streaming down my face, but close enough I could keep an eye on you to ensure your chest was still rising and falling with each breath.

The tears came because I get defeated too. I get scared too. My heart breaks too. My spirit breaks for you and all the difficulties you face. It is not fair you have to face them due to something that is due to a random change in your genetic code.

I didn't want you to see that I feel defeated too. I wanted you to know that you had a rock beside you. But sometimes there are such large forces so large in the HAE world that they can break rocks. Sometimes, nothing can be strong enough to hold the rock together in the face of such pain and the terror in your eyes.

Then I heard your determination to get up and face the world with the strength you can collect up from the tiny bits HAE has shattered all around you. It is then that I know I must do the same.

So, I dry my tears. I put a smile on my bravest face, and prepare to march forward again with you today.

From,

Also Determined HAE Caregiver

Dear HAE,

I've become accustomed to the range of emotions you conjure in me; but there will always be some rare conflicting emotions that will forever lack explanation.

Self-infusion will always be one of those areas where conflicting emotions rise to the surface.

Each time I sit down to do an infusion, I attempt to put an energy of gratefulness into the universe for the sense of personal empowerment that self-infusion has provided me with. Many professionals advocated for me to finally gain permission to access treatment in this manner and I am grateful.

But it is never that easy.

Instead, the feeling of gratitude is mixed with so many feelings that bubble to the surface:

- Anger at my genetic code for requiring me to have to learn self-infusion at all.

- Frustration at the lack of understanding in many healthcare settings for the need and importance of self-infusion.

- Fear for those that I know in the HAE community that are still fighting in their respective healthcare communities to have access to home infusion.

- Anxiety about planning daily life and travel around finding appropriate spaces to do self-infusion with my well-used and difficult veins that are weary after a decade of daily pokes.

Despite all these other emotions, I know I need to increase my feelings of gratitude to allow them to overpower the negative emotions.

So, I press on the best way I know how: with a deep breath, a smile on my face, and another IV poke for today that will allow a life-giving treatment to flow through my veins.

From,

The Emotional HAE Patient

Dear Emotional HAE Patient,

After helping you with your infusion, I marvel at our commonality. I also experience mixed emotions bubbling to the surface when it comes to home infusions.

After fighting many health care systems for several years to gain both the privilege and responsibility for home infusion, gratitude is what should fill us up.

And it does! I do have much gratitude for the freedom to infuse at home and have such timely access to a treatment that helps you live a better life.

But I also have many other mixed emotions swirling around with that gratitude.

Like you, I have anger, fear, frustration, and anxiety all mixed in with that gratitude. On top of it all, I have guilt for feeling anything but grateful when it comes to home infusions.

I make jokes as we sit together and infuse. I give your veins silly names, I make up silly songs as we infuse, and we blast music to distract us from the reality of what we're doing.

Life can change in an instant without home infusion. We have both become masters at doing anything we can to distract ourselves from the reality of home infusion and this life-threatening disease.

Regardless of the distractions, the reality of learning to give you an IV often fills me. The reality that I do this to help control what seems so uncontrollable. The reality that I do this to help keep you alive. The reality that is often so surreal that if I don't use humour, I don't know how to sit comfortably in the depths of this dark place HAE so often puts us in.

So, as you so wisely have taught me, all we can do for today with such complex emotions is take another breath, do another poke, and press on as best as we can for today.

Let's carry on together.

From,

The Also Emotional HAE Caregiver

Dear HAE,

There have been many medical textbooks, websites, journal articles, and brochures I have read with an explanation what you are. They say you are episodic, and that a patient can resolve each attack with appropriate medications and carry on with their life as usual.

While that explanation is a summary of some parts of this disease, it does little to explain what it is like to live with the trauma of this disease every day.

It doesn't explain what it is like to live with you every day, HAE: with the trauma of having attacks bring you so close to death, of the uncertainty, of wondering if I will succumb to that call of death or defeat it. The outcome is ultimately outside of my control once the swell begins.

That explanation does little to explain the mesh of trauma that floats around in my head:

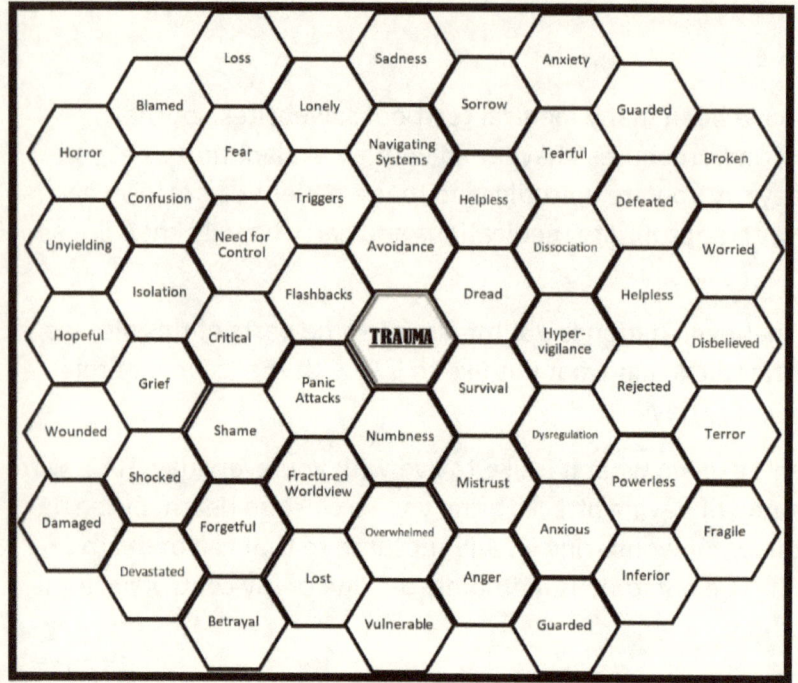

When the daily trauma of living with the disease is recognized, it becomes understood that this disease affects a whole person and needs interventions that address the whole person in order to live well.

From,

The Traumatized HAE Patient

Dear Traumatized HAE Patient,

Please know I see it. The trauma of living with HAE. It is all around us. Both of us. Every day in so many ways.

I truly do see it.

I feel it.

I witness it.

I sit in the terror of it with you.

I believe you in every moment of every day when you share how terrified you are.

I see others witness it and dismiss it as requiring you to have better "stress management."

I see others with their whispers that you are "faking it" and that it "can't really be that bad."

I want to tell others there is no way that you can be "faking it." If you are faking anything, it is being well and trying to live a life without the constraints of this disease!

I want to take it all away for you.

But I know I can't.

I know it is impossible to live somewhere between life and death and not have trauma immensely impact you.

It impacts me immensely too.

To witness you struggle so much to breathe adds to my trauma.

To witness medical professionals just dismiss you, whether out of ignorance or ego, adds to my trauma.

To witness your spirit, go from being so alive as I know you to be, to being near death adds to my trauma.

To watch you feel powerless immersed in so many systems adds to my trauma.

Trauma doesn't play fair. It doesn't help us survive HAE any better.

But I know healing from trauma is possible.

I know this because I see it in your eyes every day. I see how far you've come. I see how you've chosen healing over trauma. I see how far you've come every day.

I will be beside you in this trauma. Always.

Please know it is never you against the trauma of HAE.

It is the trauma of HAE against BOTH of us.

Please don't sit alone in your trauma.

Let's label it.

Let's talk about it.

Let's take away its power to bring us fear.

Let's rise above it together.

From,

Also Traumatized HAE Caregiver

HAE Toolkit for Living a Life of Trauma and Ultra-Rare Disease

Toolkit for HAE Patients

1. Know that it is perfectly acceptable to say, "I'm not okay. I need help coping."
2. When help is offered, be open to accepting that help. Willingness to accept help is an exercise in vulnerability, especially when the help offered may not be perfect at first.
3. Find a therapist that truly understands all trauma at its core, preferably one that is trained in Eye Movement Desensitization and Reprocessing (EMDR). Ensure they appreciate how your medical trauma shatters four key understandings: your basic worldview and/or spiritual beliefs; the belief that the world is a safe place; the belief that all is okay; and that you are worthy of feeling safe.
4. Create a box of coping cards. On one side of the card, write down what you know to be the most terrifying or challenging situations you deal with in relation to your HAE. On the other side, list anything and everything that helps you remember what to do to make it through those difficult moments such as: coping strategies; contact information for supportive individuals and professionals; helpful quotes; images that foster belief in the fluidity of hope; books to read; artwork; photographs of moments of progress to remember; and any other supports. Then, pull out the cards in those hard moments. Use them when you are sure you cannot possibly make it through another day surrounded by the challenges that come with living with HAE. Keep them where you know you might need them the most, such as by your infusion or treatment supplies.
5. Have handy a list of things that can help ground you when you feel increased distress around a swell. Include on your list: helpful body movements; deep breathing strategies; grounding techniques that work from each of the five senses; supports readily available to reach out to; self-care techniques that work in immediate moments; and strategies for naming and releasing the strong

emotions that arise in that moment.

6. Keep a journal so you can look back and have the small moments of hope documented to help remind you more of these moments will be coming.

7. When you have nothing left to give, and don't know where to turn, simply stop and pause the trauma circling around you. Gently breathe in. Then out. Know that this hard place is just one moment. The next moment may be where hope will triumph over the challenges of HAE. Trust that this type of moment is coming soon, keep a close watch for it to emerge when you least expect it.

Toolkit for HAE Caregivers

1. Share your worst fears with the patient and their medical team. Perhaps share what it looks like to watch them in ICU, hoping they will wake up, or what it looks like see the patient near death struggling with those last few breaths before they are intubated. Don't avoid the hard truths of talking about the trauma that comes with HAE. Avoiding them only makes the trauma worse. Labelling it in conversation helps both patients and caregivers have power over their trauma experiences.

2. Know that the needs of the HAE patient going through trauma don't trump your own. Both your own needs and the patient's needs are equally important. It is okay to seek support for both of you. You can't help the HAE patient if you are not okay yourself.

3. Release any guilt you may be carrying for spending time on yourself. This guilt will not help you find balance. Taking care of the traumatic impact of HAE on yourself first will always help you be more present to support the HAE patient.

4. Speak with the patient to find out how best to be their voice when they cannot speak for themselves. So many professionals and systems take away the patient's voice; ensure you know how to add their voice, not silence it.

5. Remind the patient as often as they need that you will be beside them through all of this, regardless of how scary this is. Tell them as many times as they need to hear it, until they really believe you. Many other individuals have left the patient in the past when HAE becomes too scary. Use both your words and your behaviours to

let them know you will not be one of those who will leave.

Toolkit for HAE Professionals

1. Be attuned to HAE patients' and caregivers' trauma responses by seeking out specific trauma-informed training to enhance your HAE specific knowledge. Use this training to inform discussions about the psychological impact of HAE on patients. Don't simply state that it must be "all in their head" or that they would cope better with "stress management techniques."

2. When providing patients with any information, consider using some basic trauma principles during each conversation such as the 3 Rs: regulate, relate, reason. In execution this looks like first helping the patient to regulate themselves to come into their window of tolerance. This is a space where they can cognitively take in information presented and tolerate their own complex emotions. Second, relate and empathize with the patient on an emotional level. Lastly, reason with them to help process the cognitive information presented to help determine complex treatment plans and next steps.

3. Consider the impact of your typical interventions and conversations with patients to examine if they may lead to possible trauma triggers. For example, encouraging a patient to take a deep breath when that patient's anxiety or panic is escalating, may seem like a suitable intervention with other disease populations. However, for HAE patients who have experienced intense trauma related to potential airway swelling and closure, deep breathing can be triggering rather than calming. Find creative ways from your trauma training to give control back to the patient when it comes to discussing deep breathing and/or consider alternative ways of grounding patients.

Section II

Grief & Loss

"You have to be grateful whenever you get to some place safe and okay, even if it turns out it wasn't quite where you were heading."
Anne Lamont

Dear HAE,

This morning, a friend tried to remind me how lucky I am because HAE is essentially an invisible illness that can only be seen if the swelling is very noticeable during an acute attack.

I was shocked to hear that others think it is only "visible" during an acute swelling attack. There was so much I wanted to say in response to that comment.

I wanted to tell her that she can see it all the time in my life, not just during an attack. However, I was too hurt and stunned to form the thoughts at the time.

I wish I would have told her that the effects of HAE are around me all the time. I wish I could have explained all the ways HAE is visible every day of my life. All one needs to do is just take a glance around my house to realize that HAE is far from an invisible illness.

A quick scan of my surroundings this morning reminded me of least 25 ways that HAE is visible all the time.

It's visible:

1. In my calendar, where there are numerous cancelled appointments and social engagements.

2. In my email inbox—I have declined many social invitations because I just don't have the strength and energy to do anything while recovering from an attack and trying to manage my fatigue.

3. In the tears of sadness, pain, and pure frustration that flow so easily during the worst of an attack.

4. In my wallet that contains a detailed medical summary sheet in case my HAE renders me unable to speak for myself with rapid airway swelling.

5. In my fridge where an entire shelf is filled with medication, and that's only enough to last me for one month since my swells are so frequent at the moment.

6. By the vomit buckets strategically placed under my bed, in my car, and on each floor of my house, in preparation for when an abdominal attack comes on.

7. On my tax return, where I've made huge medical claims for supplies, hospital parking, and so many different types of medical fees required to keep me alive.

8. In the darting of my eyes as I search a public venue to seek out a private space to start an IV for an infusion should I have an attack come on quickly.

9. When I am questioned about my medication at airport security: First, public embarrassment in front of strangers in the main security line; then, in the "special" security line as they call my physician's office to verify what it already says on the travel letter right in front of them.

10. From a quick scan of the contacts list in my phone. It reveals an equal number of medical offices as family and friend contacts.

11. On my phone where the apps called "Calm Keeper" and "Meditations for Pain" help me breathe and manage anxiety during a HAE swell.

12. In the stack of HAE information papers in my office that I take with me to each medical appointment to ensure each physician will listen to the seriousness of HAE and view the rest of my medical concerns within that context.

13. On my numerous Facebook updates from online education/support/sharing groups to help me feel less isolated, find hope, and learn from other patients across the world.

14. In the way I carefully read the face of someone who asks, "how are you doing?" before I provide a true answer and begin sharing what it's really like to walk in my shoes.

15. In my carefully organized medical file that includes documents that are generally reserved for those much older than me. They express my end-of-life wishes and entail who will speak for me should a HAE swell reach that final point.

16. In my fridge with healthy snacks that were prepared when I had some extra energy between swells, because if I don't take that time, they won't be prepared at all and my health will suffer further.

17. On my computer with files filled with tracking logs of my medications, symptoms, attacks, and infusions. All to be submitted on a regular basis to my medical team to ensure I continue to receive the medication I desperately need to save my life.

18. On my work timesheet, showing far more sick days than I would like to be recording. HAE makes it impossible to work.

19. From the stack of obituaries of HAE patients taken from this world far too soon. The grief I feel over each one helps remind me to keep fighting, keep advocating, and keep finding hope each day.

20. In my vacation planner where I assign a few days each year to try to attend HAE conferences so I can keep up to date on the latest information and research on this disease to ensure I can be a strong advocate for my health.

21. In my music playlists, based on different impacts of HAE: calming playlists to help when an attack is coming on, playlists that energize, playlists that and provide hope while I'm recovering from a swell and desperately want to return to usual routines.

22. In my growing pile of laundry, my bathroom that needs cleaning, and a lawn that needs cutting because I have other pressing needs to take care of. I know if I do it all I will bring on an attack. So, it will have to wait until another day.

23. By viewing the many cupboards filled with syringes, mix-to-mix vials, butterfly needles, and other medical supplies needed the instant a swell surfaces to do an infusion.

24. By looking at the calendar for my family on the fridge that highlights my commitments with overwhelming number of medical appointments that differs greatly from all the other members of my family.

25. By the degrees that hang on my wall that mark concrete achievements made possible by being granted disability accommodations in the post-secondary world.

While I didn't report any of these "visible" signs to my friend, I wish to say them now to help others understand that HAE doesn't just exist in the moment of the swell.

From,

The Invisible HAE Patient

Dear Invisible HAE Patient,

I hear and see your struggle with your "invisible" illness as well. I would echo all the thoughts in your letter to those who think that this disease is simply invisible.

As someone who walks beside you daily, I see more than you might think I do. I also see a few ways that HAE is visible in your life:

1. In the ways that you always respond with kindness and education about HAE. Rather than having hatred for those who do not and cannot fully understand what living a life with HAE is like, you've chosen to live a life of kindness toward others.

2. In the ways you carefully consider an invitation to an optional social engagement. In how you adjust everything in everyday leading up to the event so that you can attempt to attend those engagements that are most important to you. I also see the effects of HAE on the tear-soaked pillow case where frustration lands as another swell comes out of nowhere, leaving you, yet again, to apologize for a last-minute cancellation.

3. In the piles of work stacked on your desk at home. I see how hard you work to catch up so that the impact of HAE is minimal to your work commitments and you can maintain integrity as a responsible employee.

4. In the ways that you set up the bathroom, with a perfect soft spot around the toilet for those never-ending nights of vomiting due to relentless abdominal swells despite everything you do to prevent them.

5. In the way the bedroom door is strategically closed for a few moments after the big disappointment of having to turn down the latest travel adventure due to HAE. I know that closed door gives sanctuary for a few moments. Behind it, you rage at this

disease and then struggle to find creative ways to pick yourself up and carry on. Because you have no choice but to keep going.

6. In the way you search job postings and pass over any that state full-time commitments are necessary with no wiggle room. I see the deep disappointment in your eyes as you settle with the thought that as much as you would love this dream job, you know that living well with HAE and working full time are just not compatible right now.

7. In the way you crumble to the floor and rage at the world when you hear of another HAE warrior who has suffered at the hands of an uneducated medical system, unable to properly handle HAE in an emergency department.

8. And, occasionally, I see it as you are curled up tight with a few silent tears as you share the news of another HAE patient who has died from this terrible disease. I am thankful that I don't have to see this very often. But when I do, this visible sign of HAE is by far the heaviest sign that it is far from invisible.

The effects of your HAE, and your never-ending determination to live your life well despite HAE, will never simply be invisible to me.

I continue to look hard and see it all around us. I also see your strength to continue to live well despite all these ways HAE circles around us. While it may be invisible to others, it is always visible to me.

Carry on, HAE warrior! You've got this, even if others fail to see what is right in front of their faces. I'm here always to ensure that you will not be invisible.

From,

Also Invisible HAE Caregiver

Dear HAE,

I searched for answers for many months after I was first diagnosed with you. I hoped that a diagnosis would finally get me out of the hospital and get back to my life and the dreams I had for my future.

I hoped that the small losses I had experienced over that past year would be the last ones that you would create for me, HAE.

I came home from the hospital and had time to digest my diagnosis, look up some very basic information, and integrate the information given to me. I hoped that my family doctor could fill in the blanks for me. I hoped that with this information I could do what was needed and get back to my life again and avoid feeling as terrible as I did in hospital.

My family doctor confirmed that I had an ultra-rare disease that only a very few people across Canada has been diagnosed with I hoped the specialist he referred me to would know what I needed to do to get my life and dreams back.

The specialist listened intently to me and my family. He told us he was not an expert in HAE but was willing to learn. I hoped that as he learned he would find the perfect intervention to get my life back.

As I returned to living my life, trying to avoid certain triggers as suggested by the specialist, I hoped that I could just go back to being normal. To forget about HAE entirely as I made a conscious effort to avoid certain triggers.

Although I did everything I could to avoid triggers for HAE, I still ended up in the hospital over and over again. Medical professional didn't know what to do with me. I hoped that perhaps there would be more research that would tell me what other triggers to avoid.

As I sat in my specialist's office for what felt like the hundredth time, I let the tears flow down my face. Feeling alone, terrified and defeated, I asked him what I needed to do to not live like this anymore. I asked if he could help me get home infusion so that I could stop living in the hospital and get back to school so I could work toward the career of my dreams.

I then wrote advocacy letter after advocacy letter to executive medical professionals and government officials pleading to be allowed to have home infusion. I hoped that someone, somewhere, would see just how much I wanted more control over my life and empower me to live well instead of a life defined by HAE.

Nearly two years later, I finally celebrated the success of my advocacy efforts. I was granted permission for home infusions. I hoped that this would give me the control over my disease and my life that I wanted.

As I began a trailblazing effort to train both myself and my husband in home infusion, I hoped that what I was learning would eventually become routine. I hoped that the awkwardness, strangeness, and difficulties that come from doing home infusions would somehow become easier.

As I got back to living a more routine life, I hoped to regain full control over my life, go back to work full time, and continue my education to reach my ultimate career.

As I went back to work full time and managed my HAE swells with home infusion, I hoped the inability to complete a full week of work without being exhausted and in pain would be temporary.

As I adjusted to my new work and school schedules, I hoped that it would just be temporary and that I could find my way back full time again when my body settled better with home infusion.

As I adjusted my employment expectations to work permanently part time, I found many creative ways to manage my HAE. I found more control of my disease with home infusion.

Through all of this, I hoped to be able to build my family and have children as my husband and I had always dreamed about.

As my husband and I faced together the seventh medical professional who looked at us with worried and defeated eyes at the prospect of a pregnancy and HAE, we hoped that adoption would be the answer to building our family.

As we sat with our adoption worker, we hoped that despite the diagnosis of HAE and its resulting impact on my life, that they would approve us for adoption so we could begin raising a family.

As we tried to find a balance between my daughter's special needs and my special medical needs, we hoped that we could manage a day-to-day balance well enough to be able to travel outside the city to take a family vacation.

As we took our first family vacation only a few hours away from home, I hoped to find places to do home infusion. I hoped all the preparations I'd made to find understanding emergency medical facilities would not be needed.

As I continue to make the most of each day I'm given, live my life with home infusion, connect with my growing family, and work in a career I love, I now know that hoping for minimal loss will never be a reality with HAE.

The tsunami of grief and loss at every stage of life will continue to hit me when I least expect it.

I know the only way to continue to manage such loss in my life is to keep choosing hope over the odds, through creatively adjusting my mindset and constantly striving to find the fluidity of hope.

Today, I continue to hope for more moments where I can continue to breathe and love my family.

When tomorrow comes, and I face new challenges, I will continue to adjust what I hope for. I will keep trying to live the best life possible.

From,

Searching for Hope HAE Patient

Dear Searching-for-Hope HAE Patient,

As I read about your determination to keep redefining hope, I want you to know that I will continue to be present with your grief and loss for as long as you need me.

Please know I truly do see the losses that you face every day.

When I first saw you experiencing losses, I wanted so desperately to just fix them for you. And there are times when I still want to do that.

But I've learned that, by the very nature of this disease being rare, not even a scientifically-based, complex medical system, can take away your grief and loss with their inept answers.

I used to be at a loss for what to do if I can't take away your grief. Then you told me you don't need me to take it away. You just need me to sit in it with you.

And so here I sit.

And sit.

And sit.

And sit.

And I'm still sitting here.

Have you finally figured out I'm not going anywhere yet?

As I sit here, know that I grieve with you. I'm scared at times to show you that I am grieving too. After all, aren't I supposed to be the strong one? I don't live in your body so I will never know what a HAE swell feels like. But my grief runs beside yours.

I know you have told me that there is no sense in comparing losses or grief, that each type of grief story is just as profound as the next.

I am trying to trust you with that. I'm trying to trust that it is okay to show you my grief as well. I'm trying to show you that grief can be a shared experience and that together we can sit in the depths of it.

Perhaps we can join together in our grief. We can call a truce on having to be "brave" and "push past the grief." I'm certain that joining together in our grief can only lead to increased healing power.

I don't promise to have all the answers as we search for the fluidity of hope within our grief.

But I do promise to be here. Always.

From,

Also Searching for Hope HAE Caregiver

Dear HAE,

I knew this day would come. By the very nature of technology in the global HAE community, I knew, one day, I would hear that one of my fellow HAE patients died.

Today was that day.

I heard about it several times throughout the day. A friend that lived half a world away, someone I had never actually met in person, someone who had the exact same genetic challenges I have, died today.

How am I supposed to process this information?

How should I feel?

How do I grieve this loss?

Who was this person to me?

Am I next?

Will my death story be the next one the HAE community hears about?

My story is so similar to this patient's. This could have easily been me. Will my family be hearing a similar announcement about me soon?

There is no possible "normal" way to feel about this loss.

Instead, there is immense sadness.

And fear.

And anger.

And a complete shattering of my worldview.

I can't integrate this loss into my mind, my heart, or my soul.

I simply hate you HAE when you force me to face this kind of loss. Being a HAE patient is tough enough without facing this added loss on top of it.

For today, I will just rage at you, HAE. And probably tomorrow too. And every day afterwards until this grief changes into something that doesn't feel so raw.

But today is not that day.

Today, I am simply sad that another resilient, amazing, determined, fighting HAE soul lost the fight. I mourn the loss of a kindred spirit whose path briefly crossed mine in this world and now is abruptly no longer here.

From,

Grieving HAE Patient

Dear Grieving HAE Patient,

Today, like you, I simply hate HAE.

I have no words when HAE takes a human life. Words cannot match this injustice.

My heart pleads: please don't let the next life HAE takes be yours.

Just please, please, please, please, please don't let it take you.

Yes, today, I simply hate HAE as well.

I simply refuse to see the good in it today and for as many days as this grief sits heavy within me.

From,

Also Grieving HAE Caregiver

HAE Toolkit for Grief and Loss

Toolkit for HAE Patients

1. Name the losses as they occur, don't let them simply pile up. You can't grieve what you can't first label. You also can't begin to find your "new normal" living with HAE if you can't first label the losses HAE takes from you.
2. Find rituals that work for your own grief process and keep creating new rituals as you need them. If you struggle with knowing what that looks like for you, seek out a therapist who can hold your grief for you while you work together to sort out which rituals will fit best for you.
3. Know that your grief and loss will ebb and flow along this journey. Lean into it and be gentle with yourself as the next tsunami of grief hits you at the most unexpected of times. It is unavoidable so don't let denial rule your grief process.
4. Let go of expectations around holidays, milestones, and other celebrations. Take the time to grieve what you anticipated these to look like. Do what you need to live as well as possible for the long haul with HAE.
5. Develop an iron-clad way of ignoring the criticism from the outside world on how you live your life with HAE. Know you are doing exactly what is best for you. Don't heed judgements from the outside world regardless how loud they seem to be.
6. Find a visual ritual to represent each loss. Add to this visual when your heart is heavy with yet another loss. Then use it to remind yourself of how many losses you've endured and survived. Sit in the knowledge that it is possible to get through yet another day with multiple losses.
7. Keep searching for the hopeful cracks that spread a little light on the grief. They will always exist, but sometimes you must look hard to find them, immensely hard! Never stop looking!

Toolkit for HAE Caregivers

1. When you struggle to know if the patient wishes to talk about their grief and suffering, or if they would rather distance themselves from it in this moment, simply ask the patient what they need. Then trust them when they tell you what that may be and follow their lead.
2. Find your own space, tribe, or rituals that help you with your unique experience of grief. When you're not sure what you need, open up a conversation with a HAE patient and/or professionals to assist you in processing your own losses. Seek out your own therapist if that feels right to help you process all areas of profound loss for you.

Toolkit for HAE Professionals

1. Encourage patients to explore their own grief journey at any point along their HAE disease trajectory. Just like more common chronic illnesses, grief can cycle with many factors; processing grief is not a one-time event.
2. Know your own grief triggers so that they do not impede your ability to sit with and be present to the grief and loss for both HAE patients and caregivers.
3. Seek out solid support networks with colleagues who are open to discussing emotional impacts and burdens of working with HAE patients. By the very nature of the small professional world of HAE, distinct boundaries with patients/families may be difficult to maintain. Find a trusted place to explore that dynamic with another professional who truly understands.
4. Identify your own weak spots in being present with grief and loss and seek out additional training in these areas and/or continue to learn from patients and caregivers as appropriate.

Section III

Partnering with Professional Supports

"When we fully show up for one another, we become witness to the truth that trials and sickness and pain are not the whole story.
There is more, so much more."
Kara Tippetts

Dear HAE,

I have another clinic appointment today. I'm grateful for everything the clinic offers me as you are not an easy disease to manage, HAE. So many challenges, so rare, such little evidence, so few answers, such a burden. Therefore, I'm grateful that I have a team of people who support me and learn with me.

Even on the best days though sometimes I have trouble explaining to my medical team what I would like them to know.

Today, that includes my wish for them to understand my experience of living in this body in several areas:

1. **I think about dying from an airway attack every time I have one**. Please don't try to minimize the severity of an attack when I am in the middle of one. It doesn't matter if I am in the emergency room surrounded by all the right medical professionals and equipment. It is still a life-threatening event that requires appropriate medical intervention and has the potential to take my life. Simply acknowledging that helps me know that you understand my suffering during a HAE swell.

2. **It will never become "easier" to cope with the more HAE swells that I have.** I may learn how to read my body better with each swell, but that doesn't mean that the swell is less of a physical and emotional trauma to my body. Please understand that swell number 101 is still just as difficult as the first one my body experienced. It is even harder to experience another swell after taking the leap to try out a new treatment. To experience a swell with a medication that has taken so long to become available for patients is always just as hard as the very first swell. Swells can also be exponential harder when I think about the huge cost of medications that treat this disease and think of the unequal access to treatment across the globe. It is never easier. Just layers of different and difficult.

3. **Please don't just tell me to manage my anxiety better**. I know anxiety contributes to my swells. I know it makes it worse for me when I'm in the middle of a HAE swell. That awareness doesn't mean I can just turn it off. A swell is not a normal sensation in the body. Regardless of how well I'm coping, some sense of anxiety will likely be present as the body as bodies are not made to ignore the sensation of stopping breathing. Please don't see me as "less than" for having anxiety in the face of a life-threatening situation. Please allow our shared human connectedness within this fear and anxiety and allow that to lead you to have compassion for me.

4. **HAE does not feel episodic to me.** While it may be described that way in the medical literature, living in this body it does not feel this way. I don't only face HAE during a swell, I think about it all the time. I must continually adjust my lifestyle, goals, plans, and dreams every day to help manage and prevent my attacks. The degree to which I focus on HAE in any given moment may fluctuate, but it never fully disappears.

5. **Trusting this medical team is difficult and takes a leap of faith**. Not just this medical team—any healthcare provider. It's not just you, it's those that have come before you. I've had many others not listen to me, dismiss me, judge me, and give me wrong diagnosis, treatment, and information. This has nearly led to unnecessary surgeries and nearly my untimely death on numerous occasions. Therefore, I have learned to be my own advocate and it will forever be difficult to simply accept information at face value. I will always feel like I need to do my own research. Trusting you requires much vulnerability on my part that perhaps you can understand. Some days that is very hard. The longer we work together, the more I promise to try to be more vulnerable. Please have patience with me as I work on that evolving trust.

6. **Please always call me by my name and see me as human being**

who is suffering. Look me in the eye when you talk to me, connect with my pain, suffering, and struggles. Give me hope. Please don't just assume that because I appear to be coping at this moment, that this particular swell is easy on me. Please also don't assume that if I appear to not be coping well, that I am having a swell because I can't manage my stress. HAE swells are hard. They just are. Your acknowledgement of that simple fact makes every part of a swell less traumatic.

7. **Travel with HAE will always be difficult**. Even if my swells are generally stable, it is still hard for me to venture into areas where I may not have access to a close medical facility. Regardless of when my last swell was, traveling is difficult. It requires much planning. It terrifies me. Travelling takes me outside of my routine and has the potential to trigger more swells. Having a swell outside of my usual environment is stressful in many ways. Creating travel plans where I can keep a regular schedule and have a safe, sterile environment for an infusion is a challenge. Travelling to where there is access to HAE knowledgeable healthcare professionals is a double challenge. And the challenges just keep increasing. Please understand this and don't minimize how difficult life is with HAE, even for something that should be pleasurable such as "holidays." And yet, please understand, I still want to be able to travel. It is a normal part of life. I desperately want to experience normal and all the world has to offer by travelling.

8. **I'm going to ask you questions that you aren't going to know how to answer.** I know that medicine and science have not caught up to fully understand everything there is to know about HAE. That is fine. It's to be expected since only a handful of patients across the globe live with this disease. But, please don't just dismiss my questions because you don't know the answer. It helps me more if you tell me you simply don't know. It also helps when you explain what you **do** know and **why** there are aspects of the disease that you don't yet know about. That understanding helps me find much

more patience when dealing with the medical system and helps me formulate other questions I may have. I do truly want to understand as much as I can to help me live my best life possible.

9. **Please don't simply discount my questions**. In particular, please don't dismiss me when I tell you about something that has worked for me and/or other HAE patients. It is clear that medicine is still trying to understand this disease more fully so please take the time to hear what I have to say. If your understanding of medicine doesn't fit with what I am telling you, that is perfectly acceptable. However, please at least take the time to fully hear my experience before judging it. This is a rare disease and I am certain that sharing knowledge of it can only help us all in the long run. You never know whose life may be saved from such challenging conversations.

10. **I need your help to put my patient experience in terms that other healthcare providers will accept**. I will often encounter much bias, stigma, ignorance, and lack of understanding in the healthcare system with this diagnosis. I only know my own patient experience and I haven't been to medical school. It is very important to me that you join with me to share my patient experience in ways the medical system can hear it. Doing so helps me seek the most appropriate medical care. I continually hold out hope that it is this process that could lead to advances in medical care for this very rare disease.

11. **Please know that I still must do the things in life that are most important to me**. I know that sometimes the things I do will bring on a swell. But I don't want to miss out on my life and all that I hold near and dear to my heart. I'm sure that you want the same for your life as well. I want to ensure that HAE does not rule my life. Therefore, I may occasionally have some dreams that mean taking risks with HAE. I would rather take the risks than simply avoid living life. So, please don't view this as my lack of compliance or misunderstanding of the disease and its effects on me. Please,

simply view this with the knowledge that your patient has hopes and dreams and has decided to not give up on all that this life has to offer.

12. I am a human being with a story, not just a statistic. Please don't just look at me and see a statistic. Please see me as a whole person. I am a dreamer. A goal setter. A loved one. A human being with feelings just like you. Please help me keep my story moving in the direction that I dream it can go.

Most days I feel like my medical team already knows these things. And for that, I'm grateful. So, today, I will soak in the gratitude for my ever-learning medical team and hope that other patients are able to have the same experience in their comprehensive care clinics around the world as well.

From,

Partnering HAE Patient

Dear Partnering HAE Patient,

I marvel at how you constantly strive to put words to your experience as a HAE patient and how you try to partner with your medical team. I'm grateful that you never give up trying to have others understand the whole person experience so that you, and all HAE patients, can be treated with dignity.

I watched you at your appointment today. I wanted to say more, to support you exactly as you needed. But I'm still learning. This is harder than you can possibly know. I wish all the professionals you encounter could read your thoughts so they would understand what you need.

I would like to add one more item to your list of wishes for professionals:

Please understand that this patient is my loved one. They are loved by so many in this world and they ARE my world. They are cherished and precious.

Please always treat them as you would treat the cherished people in your own world. Please don't simply dismiss or judge this patient and their experience because they inherited a disease that you may not understand. Please treat them the same way you would treat a patient with a more commonly understood and less rare condition.

The life of this patient, and the lives of their loved ones, depend on it.

From,

Also Partnering HAE Caregiver

Dear HAE,

You have brought numerous healthcare professionals into my life. Each one has taught me a lesson that I will always carry with me.

Today, I carry immense gratitude for the wonderful compassion shown me by one particular nurse.

For her, it was probably just another ordinary day. She likely is so filled with compassion that it just comes out of her naturally. However, she made a world of difference to me, far more than she will ever know as I endured, yet again, another invasive medical procedure as a result of what you have done to my body, HAE.

I sat in the waiting room dressed in the appropriate patient attire—gown, housecoat, hospital slippers—and silently recited what I would need to tell this particular medical team.

I was prepared to let the nurse know that I had a very rare medical condition which makes doing this standard medical procedure much more complicated. This procedure had a high likelihood of triggering a life-threatening attack that would require specialized medical treatment. There could be a high chance that my life would be at risk simply because of all the unknowns related to my disease. Too many times in the past, when the medical team thought they knew better and did not listen, their actions placed me in life-threatening medical distress while undergoing a standard medical procedure similar to this one.

Before I could finish mentally rehearsing what I needed to say, this nurse called me from the waiting room. She greeted me and asked for the proper pronunciation of my name. Then, she assisted me with getting settled in the procedure room and clarified several important points: her name, her role, and a good overview of what was to happen over the next few hours.

Then, as expected, she began taking my medical history. As it came time to discuss my medical condition, I began to speak quickly, prepared to hand over the stack of medical journals and letters from my specialty clinic. I attempted to dump as much medical information about HAE in the short time allotted to take my medical history.

However, the nurse stopped me and said the perfect words I needed to hear:

> *"I have never heard of that condition before. My years of experience as a nurse have taught me that those living with rare conditions know their body, and their disease, better than anyone. Can you please tell me all that you think is important for me to know before we start this procedure? You can take as long as you need to explain it."*

With each of her words, I took deeper and deeper breaths, and relaxed. I explained how my disease would impact the medical procedure. She listened intently, only interrupting to ask questions to help her understand better.

Once I felt the nurse had a good understanding of how HAE would affect my medical procedure, she gathered the rest of the medical team around me and brought them to silence around me. She gently told them I had a rare disease and then allowed me the opportunity to tell them what I had shared with her. She didn't rush me; I had all the time I needed to ensure the team around me understood exactly what I needed them to know about HAE.

When all the questions from the team had been answered, the nurse allowed me a few moments of silence. She then asked if there was anything else I needed to shared with the team; both about my medical history and about me as a person.

I easily responded, "No, you have provided me an opportunity to share all that I need to. Thank you."

What a rare gift it was to be able to say that! The opportunity to ensure all in the room knew how to prevent me from experiencing a life-threatening situation was huge for me along this medical journey.

As the procedure began, I couldn't see what was happening, so the nurse explained each step right before the doctor did it. During the first big painful pinch, she asked me how I was feeling.

"Anxious," I replied, feeling comfortable enough to tell the truth.

She pulled up a chair, took my hand, looked me in the eyes, and told me I could squeeze her hand as hard as I needed to. Then, she continued to explain what was happening, allowing equal time for explanation and quiet time while she continued to look directly into my eyes. She did not shy away from my distress, pain, and fear.

And then it was all over. I had made it through. And it all went okay.

There are only two words that truly reflect my inner state of gratitude for such kindness: Thank you!

From,

The Grateful HAE Patient

Dear Grateful HAE Patient,

Thank you for teaching me what being present with your experience looks like. When you share what others are doing for you, it helps me know how to be present with your experience as well.

Please keep sharing, I need to keep learning!

From,

Also Grateful HAE Caregiver

Dear HAE,

Today is like so many other days as I walk through the door of yet another medical specialty office.

I know the drill: check-in, confirm my basic demographic information, have a seat, and fill out the intake form. I do it all on automatic pilot.

As I sit on the predictably hard, waiting room chair, I take a minute to do a short mindfulness exercise before putting pen to paper to fill out the intake form.

On the surface, the intake form looks like a simple two-page form with various blanks and boxes; however, for me, completing it is the equivalent of running a marathon. In fact, each time I go to complete such a form or engage in a medical discussion, I know that exhaustion will hit.

In fact, I know it so well that it's been given a name.

Vulnerability Exhaustion.

Vulnerability exhaustion creeps up in nearly every medical setting I experience. It is the exhaustion that comes from having to tell a complex, traumatic, and very rare health narrative over and over to medical professionals that do not always receive it in the most therapeutic and non-judgmental manner.

No medical question is ever as simple as it seems. "Number of prior hospitalizations?" seems to require a simple, concrete number. But what that number doesn't capture is the trauma behind each of those visits.

It doesn't capture the fear I felt in one of those hospitalizations when I couldn't speak for myself and the nurse refused to allow me to call my sister to come and advocate for me so that I could get the care I needed to safe my life.

It doesn't capture the terror that comes with a hospital stay that had such significant trauma associated with it that I only recall small snippets of the entire week's stay.

It doesn't capture the feeling of being dismissed during a hospital stay when I heard the medical team talking outside my door about how they believed me to be lying about the severity of my disease. This same team had to intubate me less than a half hour later as the airway swell predictability did not pass without medical intervention.

It doesn't capture the time four physicians all asked me what I was allergic to and why I hadn't had my EpiPen with me so I could have avoided this hospitalization. It also didn't capture the way they refused to come back to speak to me after realizing that an EpiPen would have done nothing to prevent my latest intubation, but perhaps them listening to me might have.

It doesn't capture the time three nurses, one right after the other, told me it was "all in my head" and I should "just learn to manage my anxiety better." I was then promptly rushed to be intubated that same hour.

It doesn't capture the time the nurse refused to listen to me as my airway was closing and I needed another infusion. Instead, she sent the psychologist to talk to me about my health anxiety

It doesn't capture the time I had to educate a new unit nurse each time I needed infusion on how to mix and administer the blood product. And by "educate" I mean have battles that lasted an hour or two and ultimately resulted in me asking to speak with the charge nurse and unit manager before getting the product properly delivered into my veins as it should be.

It doesn't capture the time I met with the unit manager before surgery to discuss my needs and past challenges while in hospital. She recommended that my husband stay with me at all times to ensure that medical staff did not make further mistakes as that is the only way for me to get the care I so desperately needed.

It doesn't capture the time I was encouraged to fall asleep so I could "get some rest for healing." I couldn't bring myself to close my eyes; I wasn't sure I would wake up in the morning, despite being surrounded by many professionals in hospital.

It doesn't capture the time I woke up in ICU to see the pure look of terror in my family member's eyes while sobbing through the words, "I thought you'd died."

Most of all, it doesn't capture the complete fear and terror of hospital stays when it is nearly impossible to rely on medical staff to keep you alive. The complete terror that comes from knowing that most people come into hospitals and can trust that staff will keep them alive. HAE patients come into hospital wondering if they can possibly advocate enough for themselves to have staff listen long enough to modify typical medical protocols with HAE needs in order to keep them alive.

This question about prior hospitalizations is just one simple question on the intake form. As I looked at the two page intake form for this new medical office, I took more deep breaths knowing that this particular level of vulnerability exhaustion will only continue to deplete me if I do not label it, take time to pay homage to it, and incorporate its effects into my fatigue and pacing plans for the day.

While many healthcare professionals do not take their patients' vulnerability exhaustion into account, it does not mean it doesn't have an impact. In fact, the lack of understanding only makes it more difficult to manage.

Therefore, today I take the steps needed for me to manage my vulnerability exhaustion. My self-preservation steps will hopefully allow me to reduce the level of vulnerability and give me courage to engage with this new healthcare specialist.

From,

Vulnerable HAE Patient

Dear Vulnerable HAE Patient,

Ah yes, vulnerability exhaustion.

I see it.

I witness it frequently.

I want so desperately to take it away for you.

But I don't know how to support you in it.

I know that you tell me your story and your experience. I know that you also tell others your story and your experience.

I had not previously considered what repeating your story over and over must be like for you. I am one person hearing your story only one time. I am also one person trying to support you and give you suggestions. However, you hear many suggestions from everyone you encounter each time you must tell your story.

I never considered how exhausting that must be when your ever so vulnerable and emotional story can be received so many ways.

It's no wonder there are times when the most terrifying parts of your story remain just with you. The impact of opening up and being vulnerable, only to be hurt at your lowest moments when others don't understand, must be profound.

So, for today, I simply ponder how best to support you in your struggle with vulnerability exhaustion.

I'm here. Let's keep talking about how I can support you in your struggle.

From,

Also Vulnerable HAE Caregiver

HAE Toolkit for Partnering with Professionals

Toolkit for HAE Patients

1. Assume that professionals are attempting to have your best interests in mind.
2. Assume that professionals are trying to help the best way they know how, despite the gaps in their HAE knowledge. Assuming the best from them allows for a solid foundation for building a good professional relationship.
3. Never hesitate to give feedback to professionals about what is working or not working, or what you need them to do differently. It is impossible to move forward if they are not aware what doesn't fit for you.
4. Talk to other HAE patients about the professionals they interact with on regular basis. Don't hold back with your questions; ask all you need to ensure the professional, the service, and the system will meet your needs. Keep asking until you are convinced that they appreciate the far-reaching psychosocial impacts of HAE on your life. Ensure they consider all aspects of care that affect your sense of dignity and safety as a patient.
5. Seek out system advocates and higher-level management when your needs are not being met by the frontline professionals in your case. You must advocate for yourself. Don't allow a particular professional or a system to silence your voice. Your health and well-being depend on it.

Toolkit for HAE Caregivers

1. Be willing to have a conversation with the patient about what your role as caregiver should look like. Don't avoid the hard conversations; get a clear picture of what the patient views as supportive when they are partnering with healthcare professionals for both regular clinic visits and in emergency situations.
2. Find ways to develop your own relationships with healthcare providers. Take the time to learn from both patients and the healthcare team about your unique role on the HAE team.

Toolkit for HAE Professionals

1. Be willing to sit with clinical ambiguity often with patients given the rare, unpredictable, and variable nature of HAE clinical presentations. Patients are often balancing both a cognitive and emotional understanding of HAE. Therefore, patients will likely go back and forth in their integration of understanding the reality of their disease. It is impossible to fully sit in the awareness of such a life-threatening disease every moment of every day. During this process, be willing to sit with clinical ambiguity rather than jumping to conclusions quickly with patients and/or caregivers.
2. Engage frequently in hope/worry dialogue to help manage the patient's trauma with HAE experiences and balance their expectations. Clearly share statements expressing your hope for the patient paired with your worries to help address uncertainty such as "I hope that you will return to your baseline number of swells per month, but I worry that might not be the case with this current treatment."
3. Help develop safe therapeutic relationships with patients and caregivers by naming emotions for patients. Validate complex medical experiences and trauma prior to engaging in complex treatment discussions with statements such as "I wish this was different" or "I wish science and medicine had more answers for you" or "I wish this wasn't so difficult and terrifying for you."
4. Do not attempt to move past intense emotions by offering patients certainty or making promises when medicine is unclear due to limited HAE evidence. Instead, simply be willing to sit in the intense emotions with patients and/or caregivers and acknowledge the helplessness inherent in having a lack of evidence bases for ultra-rare diseases such as HAE.
5. Be willing to explore your role within the medical team. Make the expectations of your role clear to all team members and patients alike. Avoid blurring boundaries and attempting to enhance your role to avoid feelings of helplessness when demands of patients exceed your capabilities.

Section IV

Isolation and Cultivating a Tribe

"The friend who can be silent with us in a moment of confusion and despair, who can stay with us in an hour of grief and bereavement, who can tolerate not knowing, not healing, not curing, that is a friend indeed."
Henri Nouwen

Dear HAE,

As I struggle with you, I've been hearing this lot lately: "How can I help? I feel helpless." It's the way others around me share their desire to take away my pain. They want to make it easier. They want to fix it.

I think I can understand that feeling. When I see those I love hurting or suffering, I want to fix it for them too. I want to take away all the difficult feelings, to protect them, to somehow shield them from whatever difficulty life is throwing at them.

After all, isn't that what friends and family are supposed to do? To find ways to make life easier, to ease burdens with love and care.

I feel the instinct to help others so strongly that I imagine it is a universal instinct. I know that others truly want to help when they ask. But when they ask me what they can do, all I'm able to mutter lately is, "I don't know."

And those words somehow just make it worse.

It isolates me. It creates another divide between me as an "HAE patient" and "others." I'm failing again because, not only am I suffering, I am cutting off other's attempts to help ease that suffering.

They ask a simple question.

And I can't even answer it.

So I started thinking hard on how to explain what truly helps in those moments. It turned out the answer was about "being" rather than "fixing."

What does this mean? What would it look like if others were able to help me in this way?

I think perhaps it could look something like:

1. Being fully in the moment. Being willing not to shrink back from the suffering. To sit with the suffering without the need to change it. Being real in that moment. Not finding ways to distract your mind from the suffering I represent right in front of you. Not minimizing the suffering in the moment. Not rushing to tell me that I am strong, or brave, or that everything will be okay in the end. Not trying to remove the intensity of the moment by telling me that there is larger purpose/plan to this pain/suffering. Or that I just have to have some faith in that plan and it will all make sense. Not reminding me that that I've been to this place before and have made it through, so I will this time as well. Rather, simply label it for what it is. Even if the same type of moment happens over and over. And then be willing to just sit with the weight of that moment. To be honest enough to say it is unfair and hard to watch. To be vulnerable enough to tell me it scares you to have to sit with me in this constant and unpredictable space between death and dying. And to be able to do that over and over again knowing that, while the moment may ebb and flow, it never truly goes away. And that such suffering will be present for me for a lifetime. In short, to be in the moment for as long as it takes, for as long as I need you to be there.

2. Reflect back living in that moment: Once you truly are okay to be in the moment, reflect back to me what you feel/think in that moment. Not to end being present, but rather to share the burden of that moment. Keep labelling what you feel/think/wish for in that moment. Not the surface things about the moment, but the very deep, life and death, part of the moment. And then allow for silence in the moment. The kind of silence that isn't lonely but rather filled with love, care, and understanding.

3. Universal understanding: Next, let me know I am not alone in this moment. While you perhaps don't share the pain/suffering of a HAE attack, I am almost certain there have been times where the world feels heavy for you too. None of us are immune, life is difficult for all of us at some point. It helps if you share your experience with me. I feel less lonely if I know that others encounter difficulties too. It makes it even less lonely if you tell me about how you meet those experiences, and where you find sources of hope. Or, how you made it through your own suffering to support others like me. Or, how your own experience can weigh on your heart every moment of every day, but that you find ways to be resilient in spite of it. Anything that helps me to know that these are universal feelings and I'm not alone.

4. Seeing beyond the suffering: And finally, among this all, please continue to see me as a person. The person who is whole despite suffering. The person whom you love and care about despite HAE. Please keep laughing with me. Make plans with me. Get mad at me when I've messed up. Tell me when I'm wrong. Forgive me. Believe in me. Push me when I need it. Be gentle with me when the world seems against me. Dream with me. Treat me just as you would if I weren't sick. Anything that helps remind me of the world that keeps on turning around me despite this pain/suffering and that I'm not that different just because I'm sick.

So, HAE, I need to find ways to help others understand the best help for me is not to try to fix me. Just "be" with me through this. That's all I have ever needed.

From,

The Being Present HAE Patient

Dear Being Present HAE Patient,

Okay, I get it now. Sit deeper in the moment with you.

Don't just tell you I will be there, show you with the deepest sense of my being that I will be there for you.

I'm trying.

Every day, I'm trying.

Please forgive me if I'm not perfect at this, I'm a work in progress too and this will take some time.

From,

Also Being Present HAE Caregiver

Dear HAE,

I wish I could find adequate words to help others understand what it is like to live in this body, each and every day. The list of what I wish others understood would include the following:

1. **"But you don't look sick" is one of the hardest statements to hear.** Please do not ask me when I will be "well" again. I have a chronic condition. It is real and it will never go away. I've gotten pretty good at putting a smile on my face and going about my life. But that doesn't mean I'm not sick. I'm sick all the time, just sometimes it sidetracks me from life more than other times. Please make no mistake about it: my illness goes with me wherever I go.

2. **Spontaneous activities will always be difficult for me.** Going anywhere requires much planning. That doesn't mean I don't want you to ask me to do activities with you. You are still important in my life and I want to be able to do things with you so please keep inviting me and including me. Even if I say "no" or have to cancel on you 15 times, please keep asking because the 16th time I may be able to say "yes."

3. **One of the best gifts you can give me is your understanding presence.** Please just sit with me in a moment of extreme pain, sadness, and suffering. Please don't simply remind me in those moments about all the other attacks that I have made it through. I know I have made it through a lot. But that reminder in the moment of an attack doesn't make it go away. It just dismisses the suffering that I'm feeling at the time. That's almost harder than the attack itself because it feels like no one understands how incredibly hard it is to be in my body in that moment.

4. **I need your help to avoid isolating.** HAE is a terrible disease that is embarrassing, scary, and painful, and makes me hard to be around most of the time. Isolating myself when I feel bad is easier

than asking for help. It doesn't take as much energy as reaching out. But isolating doesn't make it better. Instead, it just makes the negatives feel much bigger. I know it is asking a lot and it isn't easy, but please don't give up on me. I need help all the time to avoid isolating when every one of my instincts says that is exactly what to do. Your presence is a gift to me and helps me cope in many ways, so please keep trying to engage with me.

5. **Please understand that I experience losses every day in different ways**. Sometimes, I can easily find ways to move on. Other times, it consumes me more than I can ever find words for. This will be a lifelong process for me. Please don't just assume that because tears have happened around one loss that they will never happen again. Therefore, please just let me feel these emotions when they come and know that this will always be a part of my life. It is not up to you to make them go away, it is up to me to face them. As life moves along, these losses hit me at different times, in different ways. I can't predict when or why I will have to face them. But it is easier to face them with you continuing to walk next to me.

6. **Asking for help is hard.** Really hard. Always. It doesn't matter how many times you tell me that you want to be there for me, I will always feel some amount of guilt over asking for help. I want to be independent; a life of needing others is not one I want to live. I am forever grateful that you want to support me, but I also resent needing the support. It is a balance that will always be difficult but please keep making it be easier to ask for help by letting me know you are there for me. I need to hear that often. I also need to know that when you offer help you are doing it out of caring deeply for me rather than simple curiosity. I'm not an object to be studied and talked about. I'm a human being that needs other caring human beings to make it through this. Find unique ways to lift me up and support me through another moment when I feel sure that I cannot make it through.

7. **Often I don't know what help I need.** Asking what you can do to help is a difficult question to answer. I know that you want to "fix" what is happening to me. But you can't. No one can. But you can walk beside me. Let me experience whatever it is that I am feeling in the moment. Tell me that you love me regardless of this disease. Simply be with whatever I am feeling and experiencing right now and don't shrink back from it no matter how terrifying it may be. On any given day, that is likely the type of help I need even if I can't always articulate it.

8. **I can't always do what I want to do**. I continually have hopes, dreams, goals, and plans. HAE has a way of preventing me from reaching them in an easy manner. But not all of them are impossible. Please have patience and help me find ways to work toward them. This may take longer, require more support, or be defined differently than usual. It's important to me to not give up on them regardless of what it takes to reach them. Please help me find hope when it becomes too elusive in the middle of a HAE attack.

9. **Please enjoy your life and all it has to offer in every moment that you can**. My own quest to modify my life to avoid attacks is hard. I WANT to be able to keep up. To do the same things you are doing. But I know I can't. Even when I know it's good for my health, it makes me sad to miss out on something. But just because I can't do it all doesn't mean I want you to miss out on life. Please don't ever miss out on all you want to do and don't feel guilty for fully engaging in these activities; living your life to its fullest is one of the best gifts you could ever give me. For you to experience all life has to offer and share those experiences and feelings with me is a highlight and a wonderful part of my life.

10. **It will always be difficult to have disruptions to my work and**

schooling. Society has set expectations and places value on education and full-time employment. Working less and/or being on disability does not fit those expectations. Even if my reduced workload is justified by my trying to live well with HAE, it's still hard to not be at work and school full time. Please just witness my feelings around this when it comes up and try not to minimize this struggle for me. Please also understand that recovering from my most severe HAE attacks can be unpredictable. This unpredictability will often result in many last-minute cancellations in all commitments of life. This frustrates me as much as it does you, please just respond to those with grace and understanding rather than judgment.

11. **My journey to this diagnosis has been complex**. It doesn't mean that all I experienced prior to my diagnosis is not important. I still had these same difficult symptoms and experiences prior to my diagnosis. That makes the journey to diagnosis equally important as the rest of my health experience. I may need to talk about it sometimes and I need you to understand it so you can know more about who I am in the present moment. Even if you have heard me talk about it before, it may be affecting me differently now, so it helps to share it with you in different ways and at different times in order to fully process it myself.

12. **It is impossible to fully explain to you what it is like to experience a swell**. I know that you want to support me during a swell. I appreciate that more than you will ever know. However, it is very difficult for someone who has never had a HAE swell to truly know what it feels like. I will try to explain as best I can, but please don't be upset with me if I can never fully explain. I'm not trying to keep it a secret. We all have those private parts of our experiences that defy language. HAE is one of those parts. The worst of a HAE attack can only be experienced; it cannot be described with words. However, please don't let that stop you from being in my life. That only leads to a spiral of isolation. Instead, please be willing to sit in

the helplessness and ambiguity of it all.

13. **I will never be able to fully tell you what will trigger an attack**. It is a cumulative effect and no two attacks are triggered in the same way. I may know some of my triggers, but there is a strong possibility that many of them will remain a mystery for my whole life. I promise to explain my triggers to you as best I can, but please don't get upset with me if I can't fully explain exactly why an attack happens at a particular point in time.

14. **No two HAE patients experience the disease in the same way.** Yes, this is genetic, so there are others in my family with the same diagnosis. No, I do not cope the same way they do. Talking to them doesn't always help. We all experience this disease in our own way, in our own time, regardless of the fact that we share a similar genetic makeup. Please just let me experience this disease as it manifests for me. Don't try to compare me with anyone else.

15. **I think about dying all the time.** I think about it during an attack. Or when I can tell an attack is coming. Or when I have to talk about being sick. Or nearly every time I take a breath and every other moment in between. Just because I made it through my last airway attack doesn't mean I will make it through the next one. I have to treat each attack as if it could be life-threatening. Please don't minimize this for me. Just be willing to sit with me and accept that this is the life I lead and these are the fears I have. It doesn't help to remind me that you don't think about this all the time. It just makes it more difficult to know that I sit with these thoughts alone most of the time.

16. **This disease is lonely.** It doesn't matter who else is around me or how many other patients I connect with across the globe. There will be times when I won't be able to explain myself and, therefore, will experience loneliness that I can't translate to others. Keep checking in with me anyway. Please find creative ways to stay in my

life regardless. Know that I'm trying the best I can and that your support means everything to me. It helps to combat a small part of this loneliness in ways that defy explanation.

Perhaps, most of all, I wish for loved ones to simply be "present" with what happens to my body/heart/mind and all the suffering that comes with this disease. That in itself is an extraordinary gift.

From,

The Ever-Complex HAE Patient

Dear Ever-Complex HAE Patient,

I'm still here with you.

Sitting with you trying to understand all that you have just shared.

Again, please be patient with me as I try hard to hear all that you are saying.

I want so many good moments for you. But I also don't want to be greedy and push you into seeking out the good and just ignore the difficulties you face every day.

I'm still learning how to support the best way possible.

Please keep trying to teach me even when I frustrate you. I'm scared too. Let's face our fears together.

From,

Also Ever-Complex HAE Caregiver

Dear HAE,

While there are many days when I fall to my knees and curse the challenges and isolation that you bring me, there are other days that I find gratitude for the human connections you have brought me.

As I went about my errands today, I crossed paths with a friend who I had not connected with in quite some time. As we approached each other in the aisle of the grocery store, we exchanged obligatory greetings, promising to "get our children together soon for a playdate."

When I caught her eye for an extra moment, I saw a look I knew all too well. It was a look I'd seen in the eyes of my loved ones when they witnessed the impact of a HAE swell on me.

I paused my mission for the moment and called her name to re-engage her. When she came closer, I took a deep breath to calm my mind and body and open my mouth to speak the questions in my heart.

"What has really been going on? How can I be support for you? I can sit in the hard places with you, regardless of what they are."

With that small nudge, her eyes filled with tears. She lowered her head and her body began to shake as the tears streamed down her face. We stood in silence, embraced in a hug until the tears diminished to smaller streams down her face and the words could slowly flow from her mouth.

She began to speak of her own medical appointments, tests, diagnosis, treatments, uncertain prognosis, and the incredible fear related to it all. As she began to apologize for being an absent friend while going through her own medical storm, I interjected.

All I needed her to hear was that she wasn't alone in her situation. I would be there through all the hard parts in the days to come, regardless of what they would look like.

As I spoke minimal words of support, I thanked you, HAE, for helping me understand the power of reciprocal connection. For showing me that through my own suffering I had the capacity and connection to sit with another and their suffering. For not backing away from deep suffering as it crossed my path.

Lessons from you, HAE, have taught me that connection means being able to sit in the fear. To really look it in the face and let it know in no uncertain terms that support is not going anywhere. That regardless of how hard this becomes, that supportive caregivers are willing to sit in the depths of the fear and not back down.

It means that for as long as the uncertainty and ongoing quest for answers within the medical community are present, supportive caregivers will be present too.

It means that supports will keep looking for ways to break the cycle of isolation by saying they will never give up being present in the fear.

It means that supports will bring their authentic self to combat the fear. That they will not hide the parts of self that the world becomes scared of so easily.

That supports will say over and over as many times as needed that they will be there always. For as long as this journey allows them to be along for the ride.

So, yet again, HAE while I wish I did not have to experience the suffering that you bring to my life, I am grateful that it has taught me how to connect with another to help them be less alone with their own suffering.

From,

The Reciprocal HAE Patient

Dear Reciprocal HAE Patient,

I've tried so hard to be there for you that I didn't even realize the need to consider a reciprocal relationship—that you could be there for me too.

I know you say not to compare stories of suffering. However, to be honest, it's difficult not to. When I think of some of my struggles, I think how small they are compared to yours; you face life and death on a regular basis. That perspective is profound for me and it can make it hard to share my struggles with you sometimes.

But I hear your plea now.

I will try to remember that a reciprocal relationship is important to you.

Again, I'm a work in progress. Please be patient with me. Please keep teaching me.

From,

The Also Reciprocal HAE Caregiver

HAE Toolkit for Isolation and Cultivating a Tribe

Toolkit for HAE Patients

1. Find other HAE patients to connect with; odds are that they are going through a similar journey. Likely, they will have a greater understanding than others when you are at rock bottom and can help pull you out. Together you can search for the fluidity of hope within the HAE experience.
2. Educate others on what they need to know about living with HAE. Don't assume they know what you need. You can't expect others to help if you don't lay out what your life is like and how they could support you in a helpful way. If it's too hard to do it in person, try a phone call or email. As HAE struggles continue to change across your lifespan, update this list and communicate the changes to your supports. They can't help if you don't make them transparent for others to understand.
3. Let go of those who can't support your world living with HAE. Some will leave regardless of how much you wish they would stay. Find a way to let them go so you can open yourself up to new emerging supportive relationships.
4. Ensure you leave space open for cultivating a tribe. This ensures you don't close the door too quickly; the ones that might not seem exactly right at first, may turn out to be immensely helpful long term supports in the most unexpected moments.
5. Find the time to connect with your partner or a spiritual friend. Use the time for connecting and grounding with another human being who shares your heart and soul. This will hold immeasurable healing powers.
6. For members of your tribe where geography is a

barrier, use technology creatively to help reduce isolation. Skype, text, send video and audio messages; In our technological age, the possibilities to nurture connections are endless. If you're not sure where to start, find the HAE Facebook group that fits your needs and begin to connect with other patients around the world.

7. Appreciate your caregivers and supporters. Know that in their weakest moments and biggest mistakes they are just trying to help you live your best life possible. They are only human. Have daily gratitude for all them. Tell them daily how much you appreciate all the small things they do for you while surrounded by the challenges of HAE.

8. Find ways to divide and conquer the daily tasks with your supporters so that you each have time to connect with your tribe as needed. It might take a while to find a rhythm, but it is necessary to finding ways of seeking supportive, nurturing relationships within your tribe.

9. Keep looking for sources of hope around you. Consider people, agencies, systems, community resources, clubs, spiritual/religious institutions and beliefs, coping strategies, and basic truths you hold from your worldview. Keep these influences close on the most difficult of days and expand as needed.

Toolkit for HAE Caregivers

1. When struggling to know how best to balance supporting a patient and allowing them their autonomy, simply ask them. Then keep asking over and over to continue to have fluid conversations around independence and autonomy.

2. When patients are struggling the most with outside judgments, share the courage and tenacity to live day after day with HAE that you see in them.

3. Help patients feel at ease with their differences by telling them how their differences make them amazing

and enhance the life you share together.

Toolkit for HAE Professionals

1. Encourage patients to seek out support networks when you notice their tendency to isolate themselves.
2. Encourage patients to bring support individuals with them to every clinic visit and be present when developing plans for emergency rooms and times of crisis.
3. Have open and fluid conversations about support networks for HAE patients. Include this in your assessments for each and every clinic visit.

Section V

Finding Hope While Living with HAE

"Hope reflects belief. Hope believes in the better, in the higher, in the possibilities. Hope rejects cynicism. People with a higher level of hope believe that even though events may not work out they will not be defeated.
Hope is the dream of the soul awake."
Anonymous

Dear HAE,

Today, I'm thinking back to the time spent in the hospital as a teenager when I was first diagnosed. I'm thinking back to the doctor who had the brilliant idea to test me for a rare disorder once he heard about my complex array of symptoms.

That doctor probably doesn't remember the day he diagnosed me.

But I do.

He arrived out of nowhere next to my hospital bed to carefully deliver my diagnosis. When he started speaking, I felt relief for a moment. Finally, after many months of unexplained symptoms, I had an explanation. He identified what was happening inside my body. He provided an answer for my pain that so many other doctors had failed to come up with.

But then he shared additional information about the disease.

It explained it was a genetic and chronic illness. It wasn't going away. He explained that the medical science of this disease was poorly understood, even internationally. He reported treatment options were virtually nonexistent. No cure existed and likely would never exist in my lifetime. Not much more was known about HAE other than what he had just shared during our five-minute conversation.

Even though his words were even and chosen with special care, I sunk further into my hospital bed with each of them. I saw the quality and quantity of my years diminish before my eyes.

Then he slipped out of my hospital room as quickly as he had arrived. I was alone. His heavy words lingered in the air as tears filled my eyes.

It has been a couple decades since that day. I now realize there was so much more he hadn't told me about living with this rare disease.

Perhaps he hadn't known at the time. Here are the seven things I wish he would have told me that day:

1. That I'd find a rare-disease community. In this community, I'm not alone. It's a community filled with physicians, nurses, allied health professionals, patient advocates, friends, supporters and many others dedicated to never giving up. Each one is committed to going far beyond obligation or expectation to help patients like me live the best quality of life possible.

2. That amazing pharmaceutical companies exist in the rare-disease community. These companies are dedicated to helping individuals with rare disorders. They understand that treatment options for rare disease are incredibly limited and are on a mission to enhance research to develop new ones. I never could have imagined I'd see the development of so many new options in just one decade. They have enhanced my quality of life in ways that constantly surprise me.

3. That HAE would make me vulnerable in the best possible way. Having something so rare, and facing the ignorance of others, taught me how to be vulnerable. By embracing this vulnerability, I have deepened my relationships, and I've felt supported in ways I never knew were possible before being diagnosed.

4. It is still possible to reach for my dreams. Sure, my dreams ebbed and flowed, changed shape and sometimes took a little longer than initially anticipated. But they didn't disappear. In fact, they are often sweeter to strive for and reach because they mean so much more than I ever thought possible.

5. That HAE would help me find a career path I love. Living in this body and experiencing all that I have with a rare disease led me to help other patients. It fills my heart every single day. I couldn't imagine a better way to spend my life than doing this work.

6. The power of hope and determination is remarkable. These two forces are key to getting through the most difficult moments. When there were times that living with this disease seemed impossible, these forces stayed with me. No rare disease diagnosis can take that away. In fact, a rare diagnosis can actually serve to strengthen these forces.

7. Most of all, he didn't tell me it was possible to live wonderfully well with this disease. Therefore, I hope that the next time he needs to deliver a rare disorder diagnosis, he may also want to share just one of these items that he didn't tell me.

Perhaps a life will depend on it.

From,

The Seeking-Hope HAE Patient

Dear Seeking-Hope HAE Patient,

I agree that there was so much more he could have said that day about living with an ultra-rare disease.

I would also add to your list that there is also a whole community of HAE professionals who are amazing because they go outside their usual roles to support patients and caregivers with this incredibly complex disease.

I see these professionals in their helplessness going above and beyond in ways that completely defy words. They stretch their scope of practice to search out medical answers while at the same time advocate within many complex systems to seek out best care for their patients.

These professionals carry a heavy burden and stretch boundaries of their professions, ethics, and healthcare systems just to help patients live as well as possible with a disease that always has more questions than answers.

There are remarkable professionals who face life and death as much as HAE patients and who help bring about an extra set of strength and hope just when it is needed most.

Yes, there is always so much more to appreciate about this rare disease community.

From,

Also Seeking Hope HAE Caregiver

Dear HAE,

I haven't really given you much thought so far today. You've been easy to forget as I go about my morning routine. I paused to notice the beautiful sunrise that filled the sky with pink. And the calm that filled the house just before everyone else rose from their slumber. And many more small moments that I use to breeze right by.

You've taught me to take in these small, seemingly insignificant moments. To love them as much as any milestone. To simply enjoy the day as it is in the present moment and take in all it has to offer. Those small moments are life's best moments and realizing this has been one of the greatest blessings you have brought to me between the swellings.

I now take in a quiet moment of gratitude and move through my day, breathing, loving my family, and seeking to be creative to live my best life possible.

From,

Living Life HAE Patient

Dear Living Life HAE Patient,

I also had a day where HAE did not consume my thoughts and feelings. I'm not sure what all we have conquered to get here. However, something in our new normal has led us here.

I, too, cherish these days.

It will all be okay. I know this as much as I know I will be here to walk beside you. Always.

From,

Also Living Life HAE Caregiver

Dear HAE,

I thought writing to you would leave me hating you. And some days I did. But mostly, I realize that, among the challenges, I am grateful for your influence on my life. If fact, it makes me want to write a love letter to you for what you have done.

I wasn't sure what to think of you when we first met. In fact, I was pretty sure I hated you in the beginning.

You came out of nowhere. I'd thought I was invincible, and you threatened my life. You took away the dreams I had all planned out. You raged for reasons I didn't understand, leaving me confused. You scared others around me. You didn't play fair. But, then you changed.

You became my teacher, especially when I was not a willing student.

Because of you, I learned that I'm a survivor. You brought your best game to try to defeat me, but you also taught me how to be stronger and more vulnerable at the same time.

Because of you, I learned that life may not be fair, but it is certainly beautiful. Each breath of it! You taught me to see so many more lovely moments in each day. Many of those would have passed unnoticed if it weren't for you.

Because of you, I have richer, deeper, and stronger relationships. I can now invite others into my experience and connect on a level that eludes words. This continually finds unexpected ways to fill me up and over. These relationships constantly teach me that isolation and loneliness are inversely proportional to being open and vulnerable with those around me.

Because of you, I learned what a true privilege it is to walk beside someone else who is suffering. Witnessing such grace, courage, optimism, determination, and creativity is good medicine for leaning into every moment that life brings.

Because of you, I learned the secret powers contained within HOPE: it is fluid and ever-present; it exists in unexpected places; it can sustain even the weariest of hearts; and it truly is at its strongest when it is given the power to exist in community.

Because of you, I learned that fear is not the strongest force that exists. Much can defeat it: hope, compassion, faith, gratitude, perseverance, openness, communication, relationships, love, determination, courage, curiosity, and simply choosing to exist in this moment and the next moment. Each of these will always defeat fear—hands down!

Because of you, I learned to pause before I judge another. You help remind me that each one of us has our own story. To ensure I honour these stories, I must mindfully employ compassion even when I don't fully know what another's story holds.

Because of you, I fully enjoy and live in this moment—this very moment. You remind me all the time that I don't know what will come in the next moment. This gift allows me to truly, deeply, passionately cherish this one. And what a grand moment it is!

So, my dear HAE, despite how we first met, I am beginning to fall in love with you and accept you as my teacher a little more each day. You have helped me to live life in a way I didn't know existed until you came along. Thank you for helping me to truly LIVE LIFE each and every moment!

From,

The Living-Well-and-Full-of-Hope HAE Patient

Final Thought to my Readers

If you enjoyed this book or found it useful, I'd be very grateful if you'd post a short review on Amazon.

Your support really does make a difference and I read all the reviews personally so I can get your feedback and make this book even better and we can begin to further conversations around the emotional and psychosocial impacts of Hereditary Angioedema.

www.ingramcontent.com/pod-product-compliance
Lightning Source LLC
Chambersburg PA
CBHW051355280526
45784CB00007B/2972